SMOOTHIES FOR GUT HEALTH

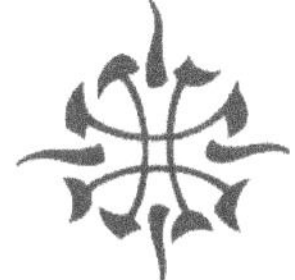

Nutritious, Easy and Delicious Recipes

Peggy C. Valentine

COPYRIGHTS

© [2024] by **Peggy C. Valentine**

TABLE OF CONTENTS

Chapter 1:

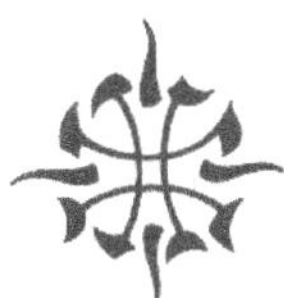

UNDERSTANDING GUT HEALTH

Introduction to Gut Health

When it comes to our overall well-being, we often focus on factors like diet, exercise, and sleep. However, there's another crucial aspect that deserves our attention: gut health. Our gut, also known as the gastrointestinal tract, is home to a complex and diverse ecosystem of microorganisms, collectively known as the gut microbiota. These microorganisms play a vital role in maintaining our health and have a profound impact on various aspects of our well-being.

The gut, which starts from the mouth and extends all the way to the rectum, is responsible for the digestion and absorption of nutrients from the food we consume. It is lined with a delicate and intricate network of cells that facilitate the breakdown and absorption of nutrients into our bloodstream. Additionally, the gut houses a staggering number of microorganisms, including bacteria, viruses, fungi, and other microbes. This collection of microorganisms is collectively referred to as the gut microbiota.

The Importance of a Healthy Gut

Having a healthy gut is of paramount importance for our overall health and well-being. A healthy gut contributes to efficient digestion, optimal nutrient absorption, and a robust immune system. On the other hand, an unhealthy gut can lead to a host of problems, including digestive disorders, nutrient deficiencies, and even systemic health issues.

One of the key roles of a healthy gut is to break down the food we consume into smaller, more easily absorbed molecules. This process begins in the mouth with the mechanical and chemical digestion of food and continues throughout the digestive tract. A healthy gut ensures that the food we eat is properly broken down, allowing for efficient absorption of nutrients and energy production.

Moreover, a significant portion of our immune system resides in the gut. The gut microbiota plays a crucial role in the development and functioning of our immune system. It helps regulate immune responses, protects against harmful pathogens, and promotes a balanced immune system. A disrupted gut microbiota can lead to an overactive or weakened immune system, increasing the risk of infections, allergies, and autoimmune disorders.

Gut Microbiota and Its Role in Digestion

The gut microbiota, comprised of trillions of microorganisms, has a profound impact on digestion and overall gut health. These microorganisms work in synergy with our own cells to break down complex carbohydrates, fiber, and other compounds that our bodies cannot digest on their own.

One of the primary functions of the gut microbiota is the fermentation of dietary fiber. Fiber, found abundantly in fruits, vegetables, and whole grains, serves as fuel for the gut microbiota. When we consume fiber, the gut bacteria break it down into short-chain fatty acids (SCFAs), such as butyrate, acetate, and propionate. These SCFAs provide energy for the cells lining the intestine and contribute to a healthy gut environment.

Additionally, the gut microbiota produces enzymes that aid in the breakdown of certain compounds, such as plant polyphenols and bile acids. This allows for better absorption of these beneficial compounds, which possess antioxidant and anti-inflammatory properties.

Furthermore, the gut microbiota helps in the synthesis of certain vitamins, such as vitamin K and B vitamins. These vitamins play essential roles in various bodily functions, including blood clotting, energy metabolism, and nerve function.

In summary, a healthy gut microbiota is crucial for optimal digestion. It assists in the breakdown of complex carbohydrates and fiber, produces beneficial compounds like short-chain fatty acids, aids in the absorption of nutrients, and contributes to the synthesis of important vitamins. By supporting the health of our gut microbiota, we can promote better digestive function and overall well-being.

Common Gut Health Issues

While maintaining a healthy gut is important, there are several common gut health issues that many people experience at some point in their lives. These issues can range from mild discomfort to more serious conditions that require medical attention. Let's explore some of the common gut health issues:

a. Irritable Bowel Syndrome (IBS): IBS is a chronic disorder that affects the large intestine. It is characterized by symptoms such as abdominal pain, bloating, gas, and changes in bowel habits. While the exact cause of IBS is unknown, factors like diet, stress, and a disrupted gut microbiota are believed to contribute to its development.

b. Gastroesophageal Reflux Disease (GERD): GERD occurs when stomach acid flows back into the esophagus, causing symptoms like heartburn, regurgitation, and difficulty swallowing. Chronic acid reflux can damage the lining of the esophagus and lead to complications if left untreated.

c. Inflammatory Bowel Disease (IBD): IBD is an umbrella term for two chronic conditions: Crohn's disease and ulcerative colitis. These conditions involve inflammation of the digestive tract and can cause symptoms such as abdominal pain, diarrhea, rectal bleeding, weight loss, and fatigue. IBD requires ongoing medical management and can have a significant impact on a person's quality of life.

d. Food intolerances and sensitivities: Some individuals may experience adverse reactions to certain foods or food components. Common examples include lactose intolerance (inability to digest lactose, a sugar found in dairy products) and gluten sensitivity (adverse reactions to gluten, a protein found in wheat and other grains). These conditions can cause digestive symptoms like bloating, gas, diarrhea, and abdominal pain.

e. Gastrointestinal infections: Infections caused by viruses, bacteria, or parasites can lead to gastrointestinal issues. Common examples include viral gastroenteritis (stomach flu), bacterial food poisoning, and parasitic infections like giardiasis. These infections can cause symptoms such as nausea, vomiting, diarrhea, abdominal cramps, and fever.

Lifestyle Factors Affecting Gut Health

Several lifestyle factors can impact the health of our gut. Making conscious choices in these areas can help promote a healthy gut environment:

a. Diet: A balanced diet rich in whole foods, including fruits, vegetables, whole grains, lean proteins, and healthy fats, can support a healthy gut. Consuming an adequate amount of dietary fiber is particularly important, as it helps nourish the gut microbiota and promotes regular bowel movements.

b. Hydration: Staying adequately hydrated is crucial for maintaining proper digestion and supporting a healthy gut. Drinking an adequate amount of water throughout the day helps keep the digestive system functioning optimally.

c. Physical activity: Regular exercise has been shown to have positive effects on gut health. Exercise can help improve digestion, reduce constipation, and promote a diverse gut microbiota. Aim for at least 150 minutes of moderate-intensity exercise per week.

d. Stress management: Chronic stress can disrupt the balance of the gut microbiota and impair digestion. Finding effective stress management techniques, such as meditation, deep breathing exercises, or engaging in hobbies, can positively impact gut health.

e. Sleep: Sufficient sleep is essential for overall health, including gut health. Poor sleep patterns and inadequate sleep have been associated with gut dysbiosis and digestive issues. Strive for 7-9 hours of quality sleep each night.

f. Avoiding excessive alcohol and tobacco: Excessive alcohol consumption and smoking can adversely affect gut health. Alcohol can disrupt the gut microbiota, while smoking has been linked to an increased risk of developing gastrointestinal disorders.

By paying attention to these lifestyle factors and making conscious choices, we can support a healthy gut and reduce the risk of gut health issues. It's important to note that if you experience persistent or severe gut health issues, it is advisable to consult with a healthcare professional for proper evaluation and guidance.

Chapter 2:

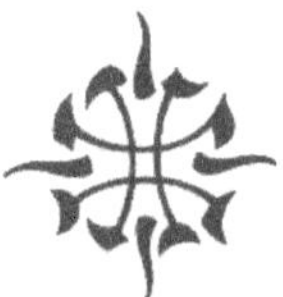

FOUNDATIONS OF GUT-HEALING SMOOTHIES

Key Ingredients for Gut Health

When it comes to promoting gut health, incorporating certain key ingredients into your diet can make a significant difference. These ingredients provide essential nutrients, support the growth of beneficial gut bacteria, and help maintain a healthy digestive system. Let's explore some of the key ingredients for gut health:

a. Fiber-rich foods: Dietary fiber is essential for a healthy gut. It helps regulate bowel movements, promotes the feeling of fullness, and serves as fuel for beneficial gut bacteria. Incorporate fiber-rich foods such as fruits, vegetables, whole grains, legumes, and seeds into your meals.

b. Fermented foods: Fermented foods are rich in probiotics, which are beneficial bacteria that support gut health. Examples of fermented foods include yogurt, kefir, sauerkraut, kimchi, and miso. These foods introduce live cultures into the gut, promoting a diverse and balanced gut microbiota.

c. Omega-3 fatty acids: Omega-3 fatty acids, found in fatty fish like salmon, mackerel, and sardines, as well as in chia seeds and flaxseeds, have anti-inflammatory properties that can benefit gut health. They help reduce inflammation in the gut and support overall digestive function.

d. Ginger and turmeric: Ginger and turmeric are known for their anti-inflammatory and digestive properties. They can help soothe the digestive tract, alleviate gastrointestinal discomfort, and promote healthy digestion. Incorporating these spices into your meals or enjoying them as herbal teas can be beneficial.

e. Bone broth: Bone broth is rich in collagen, gelatin, and amino acids that support gut health. These components help repair and strengthen the gut lining, reducing inflammation and supporting optimal digestion. You can make your own bone broth using bones from poultry, beef, or fish.

f. Green leafy vegetables: Green leafy vegetables like spinach, kale, and Swiss chard are packed with nutrients and fiber. They provide essential vitamins, minerals, and antioxidants that support gut health and overall well-being.

Remember, a balanced and varied diet that includes a combination of these key ingredients is essential for promoting gut health. Be sure to consult with a healthcare professional or registered dietitian for personalized recommendations based on your specific dietary needs and health goals.

Superfoods and Their Benefits

The term "superfoods" has gained popularity in recent years, referring to nutrient-dense foods that offer numerous health benefits. While there is no strict definition of superfoods, incorporating them into your diet can provide a wide range of nutrients and support overall well-being. Let's explore some superfoods and their benefits:

a. Blueberries: Blueberries are rich in antioxidants, particularly anthocyanins, which have been associated with numerous health benefits. They help reduce oxidative stress, support brain health, and promote a healthy cardiovascular system. Blueberries are also a good source of fiber and vitamins C and K.

b. Avocado: Avocados are packed with healthy monounsaturated fats, which can help reduce inflammation and support heart health. They are also a great source of fiber, vitamins, and minerals, including potassium, vitamin K, vitamin E, and B vitamins.

c. Kale: Kale is a nutrient powerhouse, loaded with vitamins A, C, and K, as well as minerals like calcium and potassium. It is also rich in antioxidants and fiber. Incorporating kale into your diet can support eye health, strengthen the immune system, and promote healthy digestion.

d. Quinoa: Quinoa is a gluten-free grain that is rich in protein, fiber, and essential amino acids. It provides a good source of carbohydrates for energy and is considered a complete protein. Quinoa is also rich in minerals like magnesium, iron, and zinc.

e. Chia seeds: Chia seeds are tiny powerhouses of nutrition. They are rich in fiber, omega-3 fatty acids, and antioxidants. When soaked, chia seeds form a gel-like consistency, which can aid in digestion and promote a feeling of fullness. They can be added to smoothies, yogurt, or used as an egg substitute in baking.

f. Greek yogurt: Greek yogurt is a protein-rich food that also provides beneficial probiotics. It supports gut health, promotes satiety, and provides essential nutrients like calcium and vitamin D. Choose plain Greek yogurt without added sugars for optimal benefits.

Incorporating a variety of superfoods into your diet can provide a wide range of nutrients and support overall health. However, it's important to remember that a balanced diet should include a variety of foods from different food groups to ensure you receive a wide spectrum of nutrients.

Prebiotics and Probiotics in Smoothies

Smoothies can be a delicious and convenient way to incorporate prebiotics and probiotics into your diet. Prebiotics are non-digestible fibers that serve as food for beneficial gut bacteria, while probiotics are live microorganisms that provide health benefits when consumed. Let's explore how you can include prebiotics and probiotics in your smoothies:

a.To incorporate prebiotics into your smoothies, you can consider adding the following ingredients:

- Bananas: Bananas are a great source of prebiotic fiber called fructooligosaccharides (FOS). They add natural sweetness and creaminess to your smoothies.

- Berries: Berries like raspberries, strawberries, and blackberries contain fiber that acts as a prebiotic and supports the growth of beneficial bacteria in the gut.

- Chicory root: Chicory root powder is a concentrated source of inulin, a prebiotic fiber. Adding a teaspoon of chicory root powder to your smoothie can provide prebiotic benefits.

- Flaxseeds: Flaxseeds are not only a source of omega-3 fatty acids but also contain prebiotic fiber. Grind flaxseeds before adding them to your smoothie for better digestion and nutrient absorption.

To incorporate probiotics into your smoothies, you have a few options:

- Yogurt: Adding a spoonful of plain yogurt or Greek yogurt to your smoothie introduces live cultures, such as Lactobacillus and Bifidobacterium, which are beneficial probiotics.

- Kefir: Kefir is a fermented milk drink that is rich in probiotics. You can use kefir as a base for your smoothie or add it directly to the mix.

- Probiotic supplements: If you have a specific probiotic supplement that you prefer, you can add the recommended dosage to your smoothie. Make sure to follow the instructions on the supplement label.

When making smoothies, it's important to consider the balance of flavors and textures. You can combine prebiotic and probiotic ingredients with other fruits, vegetables, and liquids of your choice. Experiment with different combinations to find the flavors that you enjoy the most.

Remember, if you're using probiotic supplements, it's a good idea to consult with a healthcare professional or registered dietitian to ensure you're choosing the right strains and dosages for your specific needs. Additionally, some probiotics are temperature-sensitive, so avoid blending them with very hot ingredients to maintain their viability.

Healing Herbs and Spices

Herbs and spices not only enhance the flavor of our meals but also offer potential healing properties. Incorporating certain herbs and spices into your diet can provide various health benefits, including supporting gut health. Here are some healing herbs and spices that you can consider:

a. Ginger: Ginger has long been used for its digestive benefits. It can help soothe an upset stomach, reduce inflammation in the gut, and alleviate gastrointestinal discomfort. Ginger can be added to smoothies, steeped in tea, or used in cooking.

b. Turmeric: Turmeric contains a compound called curcumin, which has potent anti-inflammatory properties. It can help reduce inflammation in the gut and support digestive health. Combining turmeric with black pepper enhances its absorption. Turmeric can be added to smoothies, used in curries, or taken as a supplement.

c. Peppermint: Peppermint has been traditionally used to relieve digestive issues such as bloating, gas, and indigestion. It has a soothing effect on the gastrointestinal tract and can help relax the muscles of the digestive system. Peppermint leaves can be steeped in hot water to make tea or added to smoothies.

d. Cinnamon: Cinnamon not only adds warmth and flavor to dishes but also offers potential health benefits. It has anti-inflammatory properties and may help regulate blood sugar levels. Cinnamon can be sprinkled on smoothies, added to oatmeal or baked goods, or incorporated into warm beverages.

e. Fennel: Fennel seeds have been used as a digestive aid for centuries. They can help relieve bloating, gas, and indigestion. Fennel seeds can be steeped in hot water to make tea or added to dishes for a mild, licorice-like flavor.

f. Chamomile: Chamomile is known for its calming properties and can help relax the digestive system. It may help relieve gastrointestinal discomfort, promote better sleep, and reduce stress levels. Chamomile can be brewed as tea and enjoyed on its own or added to smoothies.

Remember, while herbs and spices can offer potential health benefits, it's important to use them in moderation and consider any specific health conditions or medications you may be taking. If you have any concerns or questions, it's best to consult with a healthcare professional or a registered dietitian.

Choosing the Right Base for Gut-Healing Smoothies

When creating gut-healing smoothies, the choice of base ingredients is crucial. The base provides the liquid and consistency for your smoothie and can contribute to its nutritional value. Here are some options for choosing the right base for gut-healing smoothies:

a. Water: Pure water is a simple and hydrating base for smoothies. It helps maintain proper hydration and ensures that the other ingredients blend smoothly. Water is a good choice if you prefer a lighter and more refreshing smoothie.

b. Coconut water: Coconut water is naturally sweet and rich in electrolytes, making it a hydrating base for smoothies. It contains potassium, which is important for maintaining proper muscle function, including the muscles of the digestive system.

c. Almond milk or other nut milks: Unsweetened almond milk or other nut milks like cashew or hazelnut milk can provide a creamy base for your smoothie. These dairy-free alternatives are lower in calories and can be a suitable option for individuals with lactose intolerance or dairy sensitivities.

d. Greek yogurt or kefir: Greek yogurt or kefir can add creaminess and provide probiotics to your smoothie. They are rich in protein and can help support gut health. Choose plain, unsweetened varieties to avoid added sugars.

e. Aloe vera juice: Aloe vera juice is known for its potential soothing effects on the digestive system. It can help reduce inflammation and support gut health. It is important to choose a high-quality, pure aloe vera juice without added sugars or additives.

f. Green tea: Brewed green tea can be a base for your smoothie, providing antioxidants and potential metabolic benefits. Green tea has been associated with improved gut health and may support digestion.

When choosing a base for your gut-healing smoothie, consider your personal preferences, dietary restrictions, and overall nutritional goals. You can also experiment with combining different bases or using a combination of water and a creamy base like yogurt or almond milk to achieve the desired consistency and flavor. Additionally, ensure that the base you choose complements the other gut-healing ingredients you plan to include in your smoothie.

Chapter 3:

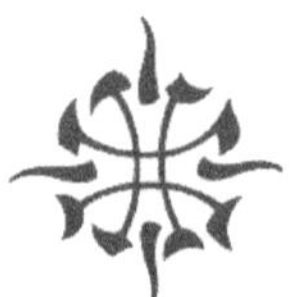

SMOOTHIES FOR DIGESTIVE SUPPORT

Banana Ginger Smoothie

Preparation time: 5 minutes

Servings: 1

Ingredients:

- 1 ripe banana

- 1-inch piece of fresh ginger, peeled and grated

- 1 cup unsweetened almond milk (or any other milk of your choice)

- 1 tablespoon honey or maple syrup (optional, for added sweetness)

- Ice cubes (optional)

Directions:

1. Peel the banana and cut it into chunks.

2. Place the banana chunks, grated ginger, almond milk, and sweetener (if using) into a blender.

3. Blend until smooth and creamy.

4. If desired, add a few ice cubes and blend again to chill the smoothie.

5. Pour into a glass and serve immediately.

Nutrition:

This smoothie is packed with potassium, fiber, and antioxidants from the banana, while the ginger provides digestive benefits and adds a spicy kick. The almond milk adds creaminess without the need for dairy. The nutritional content may vary based on the specific ingredients and optional sweetener used.

Papaya Mint Smoothie

Preparation time: 10 minutes

Servings: 2

Ingredients:

- 1 ripe papaya, peeled, seeded, and cubed

- 1 cup coconut water

- 1/2 cup fresh mint leaves

- Juice of 1 lime

- 1 tablespoon honey or agave syrup (optional, for added sweetness)

- Ice cubes

Directions:

1. In a blender, combine the papaya cubes, coconut water, mint leaves, lime juice, and sweetener (if using).

2. Blend until smooth and well combined.

3. Add a few ice cubes and blend again to chill the smoothie.

4. Pour into glasses and garnish with additional mint leaves, if desired.

5. Serve immediately.

Nutrition:

This refreshing smoothie is rich in vitamin C, fiber, and digestive enzymes from the papaya. The mint provides a cooling effect and adds a burst of freshness. Coconut water offers hydration and electrolytes. The nutritional content may vary based on the specific ingredients and optional sweetener used.

Pineapple Cucumber Smoothie

Preparation time: 5 minutes

Servings: 1

Ingredients:

- 1 cup chopped pineapple

- 1/2 cucumber, peeled and chopped

- 1 cup coconut water or water

- Juice of 1 lime

- A handful of spinach leaves (optional, for added nutrients)

- Ice cubes

Directions:

1. Place the chopped pineapple, cucumber, coconut water or water, lime juice, and spinach leaves (if using) into a blender.

2. Blend until smooth and well combined.

3. Add a few ice cubes and blend again to chill the smoothie.

4. Pour into a glass and serve immediately.

Nutrition:

This tropical smoothie combines the sweetness of pineapple with the refreshing taste of cucumber. Pineapple is a good source of vitamin C and bromelain, an enzyme known for its anti-inflammatory properties. Cucumber adds hydration and a boost of vitamins and minerals. Spinach leaves can be added for an extra nutrient boost. The nutritional content may vary based on the specific ingredients used.

Kiwi Spinach Smoothie

Preparation time: 5 minutes

Servings: 1

Ingredients:

- 2 ripe kiwis, peeled and sliced

- 1 cup fresh spinach leaves

- 1/2 cup plain Greek yogurt

- 1 tablespoon honey or maple syrup (optional, for added sweetness)

- 1/2 cup almond milk or any other milk of your choice

- Ice cubes

Directions:

1. Place the sliced kiwis, spinach leaves, Greek yogurt, sweetener (if using), almond milk, and ice cubes into a blender.

2. Blend until smooth and creamy.

3. Add more almond milk if needed to achieve the desired consistency.

4. Pour into a glass and serve immediately.

Nutrition:

This vibrant green smoothie is packed with vitamin C, fiber, and antioxidants from the kiwis. Spinach adds iron, folate, and additional vitamins. Greek yogurt provides protein and probiotics for gut health. The almond milk adds creaminess. The nutritional content may vary based on the specific ingredients and optional sweetener used.

Blueberry Aloe Vera Smoothie

Preparation time: 5 minutes

Servings: 1

Ingredients:

- 1 cup frozen blueberries

- 1/2 cup aloe vera juice (pure and unsweetened)

- 1/2 cup coconut water or water

- 1 tablespoon chia seeds

- 1 tablespoon honey or agave syrup (optional, for added sweetness)

- Ice cubes

Directions:

1. In a blender, combine the frozen blueberries, aloe vera juice, coconut water or water, chia seeds, and sweetener (if using).

2. Blend until smooth and well combined.

3. Add a few ice cubes and blend again to chill the smoothie.

4. Pour into a glass and serve immediately.

Nutrition:

This smoothie is rich in antioxidants, fiber, and vitamin C from the kiwis. Spinach adds iron, calcium, and additional vitamins. Greek yogurt provides protein and probiotics, while almond milk adds creaminess. The nutritional content may vary based on the specific ingredients and optional sweetener used.

4. Pour into a glass and serve immediately.

Nutrition:

This antioxidant-rich smoothie combines the goodness of blueberries with the potential soothing effects of aloe vera. Blueberries are packed with vitamins, minerals, and fiber. Aloe vera juice may help support gut health and reduce inflammation. Chia seeds add omega-3 fatty acids and additional fiber. The nutritional content may vary based on the specific ingredients and optional sweetener used.

Mango Turmeric Smoothie

Preparation time: 5 minutes

Servings: 1

Ingredients:

- 1 ripe mango, peeled and diced

- 1/2 teaspoon ground turmeric

- 1/2 cup coconut milk (or any other milk of your choice)

- 1/2 cup plain Greek yogurt

- 1 tablespoon honey or maple syrup (optional, for added sweetness)

- Ice cubes

Directions:

1. Place the diced mango, ground turmeric, coconut milk, Greek yogurt, and sweetener (if using) into a blender.

2. Blend until smooth and creamy.

3. Add a few ice cubes and blend again to chill the smoothie.

4. Pour into a glass and serve immediately.

Nutrition:

This smoothie combines the tropical sweetness of mango with the anti-inflammatory properties of turmeric. Mango is rich in vitamins A and C, while turmeric adds a vibrant color and potential health benefits. Coconut milk and Greek yogurt provide creaminess and protein. The nutritional content may vary based on the specific ingredients and optional sweetener used.

Orange Carrot Ginger Smoothie

Preparation time: 5 minutes

Servings: 1

Ingredients:

- 1 large orange, peeled and segmented

- 1 medium carrot, peeled and chopped

- 1-inch piece of fresh ginger, peeled and grated

- 1/2 cup coconut water or water

- 1 tablespoon honey or agave syrup (optional, for added sweetness)

- Ice cubes

Directions:

1. In a blender, combine the orange segments, chopped carrot, grated ginger, coconut water or water, and sweetener (if using).

2. Blend until smooth and well combined.

3. Add a few ice cubes and blend again to chill the smoothie.

4. Pour into a glass and serve immediately.

Nutrition:

This vibrant orange smoothie is packed with vitamin C and beta-carotene from the orange and carrot. Ginger adds a spicy kick and potential digestive benefits. Coconut water provides hydration and electrolytes. The nutritional content may vary based on the specific ingredients and optional sweetener used.

Watermelon Mint Smoothie

Preparation time: 5 minutes

Servings: 1

Ingredients:

- 2 cups seedless watermelon, cubed

- 1 tablespoon fresh mint leaves

- Juice of 1 lime

- 1/2 cup coconut water or water

- Ice cubes

Directions:

1. Place the watermelon cubes, mint leaves, lime juice, and coconut water or water into a blender.

2. Blend until smooth and well combined.

3. Add a few ice cubes and blend again to chill the smoothie.

4. Pour into a glass and serve immediately.

Nutrition:

This refreshing smoothie is perfect for hot summer days. Watermelon is hydrating and rich in vitamins A and C. Mint adds a cooling effect and freshness. Lime juice adds a tangy flavor. Coconut water provides hydration and electrolytes. The nutritional content may vary based on the specific ingredients used.

Strawberry Basil Smoothie

Preparation time: 5 minutes

Servings: 1

Ingredients:

- 1 cup fresh or frozen strawberries

- 4-5 fresh basil leaves

- 1/2 cup plain Greek yogurt

- 1/2 cup almond milk or any other milk of your choice

- 1 tablespoon honey or maple syrup (optional, for added sweetness)

- Ice cubes

Directions:

1. In a blender, combine the strawberries, basil leaves, Greek yogurt, almond milk, and sweetener (if using).

2. Blend until smooth and well combined.

3. Add a few ice cubes and blend again to chill the smoothie.

4. Pour into a glass and serve immediately.

Nutrition:

This delightful smoothie combines the sweetness of strawberries with the aromatic flavor of basil. Strawberries are rich in vitamin C and antioxidants. Basil adds a unique twist and potential health benefits. Greek yogurt provides protein and creaminess. The nutritional content may vary based on the specific ingredients and optional sweetener used.

Pear Celery Cilantro Smoothie

Preparation time: 5 minutes

Servings: 1

Ingredients:

- 1 ripe pear, cored and chopped

- 1 stalk celery, chopped

- 1/4 cup fresh cilantro leaves

- Juice of 1 lime

- 1/2 cup coconut water or water

- Ice cubes

Directions:

1. Place the chopped pear, celery, cilantro leaves, lime juice, and coconut water or water into a blender.

2. Blend until smooth and well combined.

3. Add a few ice cubes and blend again to chill the smoothie.

4. Pour into a glass and serve immediately.

Nutrition:

This smoothie combines the sweetness of pear with the refreshing taste of celery and the unique flavor of cilantro. Pears are a good source of fiber and vitamin C. Celery adds hydration and provides vitamins and mineralssuch as vitamin K and potassium. Cilantro adds a burst of freshness and potential detoxifying properties. The nutritional content may vary based on the specific ingredients used.

Green Apple Kale Smoothie

Preparation time: 5 minutes

Servings: 1

Ingredients:

- 1 green apple, cored and chopped

- 1 cup chopped kale leaves (stems removed)

- 1/2 cup cucumber, chopped

- 1/2 cup coconut water or water

- Juice of 1 lemon

- 1 tablespoon honey or agave syrup (optional, for added sweetness)

- Ice cubes

Directions:

1. Place the chopped green apple, kale leaves, cucumber, coconut water or water, lemon juice, and sweetener (if using) into a blender.

2. Blend until smooth and well combined.

3. Add a few ice cubes and blend again to chill the smoothie.

4. Pour into a glass and serve immediately.

Nutrition:

This green smoothie is packed with vitamins, minerals, and fiber. Green apples provide a tart and crisp flavor while kale adds nutritional benefits such as vitamin K and antioxidants. Cucumber adds hydration and a refreshing taste. Lemon juice adds tanginess. The nutritional content may vary based on the specific ingredients and optional sweetener used.

Avocado Lime Smoothie

Preparation time: 5 minutes

Servings: 1

Ingredients:

- 1 ripe avocado, peeled and pitted

- Juice of 2 limes

- 1 cup almond milk or any other milk of your choice

- 1 tablespoon honey or maple syrup (optional, for added sweetness)

- Ice cubes

Directions:

1. In a blender, combine the ripe avocado, lime juice, almond milk, and sweetener (if using).

2. Blend until smooth and creamy.

3. Add a few ice cubes and blend again to chill the smoothie.

4. Pour into a glass and serve immediately.

Nutrition:

This smoothie combines the creaminess of avocado with the tanginess of lime. Avocado provides healthy fats, fiber, and various vitamins and minerals. Lime adds a refreshing and citrusy twist. Almond milk adds creaminess without dairy. The nutritional content may vary based on the specific ingredients and optional sweetener used.

Raspberry Chia Seed Smoothie

Preparation time: 5 minutes

Servings: 1

Ingredients:

- 1 cup frozen raspberries

- 1 tablespoon chia seeds

- 1 cup almond milk or any other milk of your choice

- 1 tablespoon honey or agave syrup (optional, for added sweetness)

- Ice cubes

Directions:

1. Place the frozen raspberries, chia seeds, almond milk, and sweetener (if using) into a blender.

2. Blend until smooth and well combined.

3. Add a few ice cubes and blend again to chill the smoothie.

4. Pour into a glass and serve immediately.

Nutrition:

This vibrant smoothie is packed with antioxidants, fiber, and omega-3 fatty acids from the raspberries and chia seeds. Raspberries are also a good source of vitamin C. Chia seeds add a gel-like texture and provide additional fiber and healthy fats. Almond milk adds creaminess. The nutritional content may vary based on the specific ingredients and optional sweetener used.

Preparation time: 5 minutes

Servings: 1

Ingredients:

- 2 ripe peaches, peeled and sliced

- 1/2-inch piece of fresh ginger, peeled and grated

- 1 cup coconut water or water

- 1 tablespoon honey or maple syrup (optional, for added sweetness)

- Ice cubes

Directions:

1. In a blender, combine the sliced peaches, grated ginger, coconut water or water, and sweetener (if using).

2. Blend until smooth and well combined.

3. Add a few ice cubes and blend again to chill the smoothie.

4. Pour into a glass and serve immediately.

Nutrition:

This smoothie combines the sweetness of peaches with the spiciness of ginger. Peaches are rich in vitamins A and C. Ginger adds potential digestive benefits and a zesty flavor. Coconut water provides hydration and electrolytes. The nutritional content may vary based on the specific ingredients and optional sweetener used.

Preparation time: 5 minutes

Servings: 1

Ingredients:

- 2 cups seedless watermelon, cubed

- 1/2 cup coconut water

- Juice of 1 lime

- 1 tablespoon honey or agave syrup (optional, for added sweetness)

- Ice cubes

Directions:

1. Place the watermelon cubes, coconut water, lime juice, and sweetener (if using) into a blender.

2. Blend until smooth and well combined.

3. Add a few ice cubes and blend again to chill the smoothie.

4. Pour into a glass and serve immediately.

Nutrition:

This refreshing smoothie combines the hydrating properties of coconut water with the sweetness of watermelon. Watermelon is rich in vitamins A and C and provides hydration. Coconut water adds electrolytes and a subtle tropical flavor. Lime juice adds a tangy twist. The nutritional content may vary based on the specific ingredients and optional sweetener used.

Preparation time: 5 minutes

Servings: 1

Ingredients:

- Juice of 1 lemon

- 1 cup fresh parsley leaves

- 1 banana, peeled

- 1 cup coconut water or water

- 1 tablespoon honey or agave syrup (optional, for added sweetness)

- Ice cubes

Directions:

1. In a blender, combine the lemon juice, parsley leaves, banana, coconut water or water, and sweetener (if using).

2. Blend until smooth and well combined.

3. Add a few ice cubes and blend again to chill the smoothie.

4. Pour into a glass and serve immediately.

Nutrition:

This green smoothie combines the tanginess of lemon with the freshness of parsley. Lemon provides vitamin C and adds a refreshing taste. Parsley is rich in vitamins A, C, and K, and adds a burst of flavor. Banana adds creaminess and natural sweetness. The nutritional content may vary based on the specific ingredients and optional sweetener used.

Spinach Pineapple Smoothie

Preparation time: 5 minutes

Servings: 1

Ingredients:

- 1 cup fresh spinach leaves

- 1 cup chopped pineapple

- 1/2 banana, peeled

- 1/2 cup coconut water or water

- 1 tablespoon chia seeds (optional)

- Ice cubes

Directions:

1. Place the spinach leaves, chopped pineapple, banana, coconut water or water, and chia seeds (if using) into a blender.

2. Blend until smooth and well combined.

3. Add a few ice cubes and blend again to chill the smoothie.

4. Pour into a glass and serve immediately.

Nutrition:

This vibrant green smoothie combines the goodness of spinach with the tropical sweetness of pineapple. Spinach is rich in iron and various vitamins. Pineapple adds vitamin C and adds a tropical flavor. Banana adds creaminess and natural sweetness. Chia seeds provide additional fiber and omega-3 fatty acids. The nutritional content may vary based on the specific ingredients used.

Plum Mint Smoothie

Preparation time: 5 minutes

Servings: 1

Ingredients:

- 2 ripe plums, pitted and chopped

- 1/4 cup fresh mint leaves

- 1/2 cup plain Greek yogurt

- 1/2 cup almond milk or any other milk of your choice

- 1 tablespoon honey or maple syrup (optional, for added sweetness)

- Ice cubes

Directions:

1. In a blender, combine the chopped plums, mint leaves, Greek yogurt, almond milk, and sweetener (if using).

2. Blend until smooth and well combined.

3. Add a few ice cubes and blend again to chill the smoothie.

4. Pour into a glass and serve immediately.

Nutrition:

This smoothie combines the sweet and juicy flavor of plums with the refreshing taste of mint. Plums are a good source of fiber and provide vitamins A and C. Mint adds a cool and invigorating flavor. Greek yogurt adds protein and creaminess. Almond milk adds a nutty taste. The nutritional content may vary based on the specific ingredients and optional sweetener used.

Beetroot Ginger Smoothie

Preparation time: 5 minutes

Servings: 1

Ingredients:

- 1 small beetroot, peeled and chopped

- 1-inch piece of fresh ginger, peeled and grated

- 1 orange, peeled and segmented

- 1/2 cup coconut water or water

- 1 tablespoon honey or agave syrup (optional, for added sweetness)

- Ice cubes

Directions:

1. Place the chopped beetroot, grated ginger, orange segments, coconut water or water, and sweetener (if using) into a blender.

2. Blend until smooth and well combined.

3. Add a few ice cubes and blend again to chill the smoothie.

4. Pour into a glass and serve immediately.

Nutrition:

This vibrant smoothie combines the earthy flavor of beetroot with the zing of ginger. Beetroot is rich in antioxidants and provides dietary fiber. Ginger adds a spicy kick and potential digestive benefits. Orange adds a citrusy taste and vitamin C. Coconut water provides hydration and electrolytes. The nutritional content may vary based on the specific ingredients and optional sweetener used.

Apricot Fennel Smoothie

Preparation time: 5 minutes

Servings: 1

Ingredients:

- 2 ripe apricots, pitted and chopped

- 1/2 cup chopped fennel bulb

- 1/2 cup plain Greek yogurt

- 1/2 cup almond milk or any other milk of your choice

- 1 tablespoon honey or maple syrup (optional, for added sweetness)

- Ice cubes

Directions:

1. In a blender, combine the chopped apricots, fennel bulb, Greek yogurt, almond milk, and sweetener (if using).

2. Blend until smooth and well combined.

3. Add a few ice cubes and blend again to chill the smoothie.

4. Pour into a glass and serve immediately.

Nutrition:

This unique smoothie combines the delicate sweetness of apricots with the mild licorice-like flavor of fennel. Apricots are a good source of vitamin A and provide dietary fiber. Fennel adds a refreshing taste and potential digestive benefits. Greek yogurt adds protein and creaminess. Almond milk adds a nutty flavor. The nutritional content may vary based on the specific ingredients and optional sweetener used.

Chapter 4:

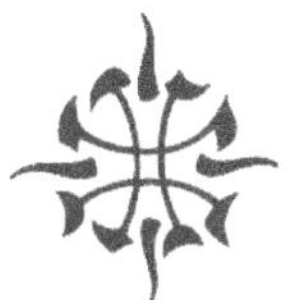

SMOOTHIES FOR GUT HEALING AND REPAIR

Papaya Coconut Smoothie

Preparation time: 5 minutes

Servings: 1

Ingredients:

- 1 cup ripe papaya, peeled and chopped

- 1/2 cup coconut milk

- 1/2 cup coconut water or water

- 1 tablespoon honey or agave syrup (optional, for added sweetness)

- Juice of 1 lime

- Ice cubes

Directions:

1. In a blender, combine the chopped papaya, coconut milk, coconut water or water, sweetener (if using), and lime juice.

2. Blend until smooth and well combined.

3. Add a few ice cubes and blend again to chill the smoothie.

4. Pour into a glass and serve immediately.

Nutrition:

This tropical smoothie combines the sweetness of papaya with the creaminess of coconut. Papaya provides vitamin C, fiber, and enzymes that aid digestion. Coconut milk adds richness and healthy fats. Coconut water provides hydration and electrolytes. Lime juice adds a tangy twist. The nutritional content may vary based on the specific ingredients and optional sweetener used.

Mango Turmeric Basil Smoothie

Preparation time: 5 minutes

Servings: 1

Ingredients:

- 1 ripe mango, peeled and chopped

- 1/2 teaspoon ground turmeric

- 4-5 fresh basil leaves

- 1 cup almond milk or any other milk of your choice

- 1 tablespoon honey or agave syrup (optional, for added sweetness)

- Ice cubes

Directions:

1. Place the chopped mango, ground turmeric, basil leaves, almond milk, and sweetener (if using) into a blender.

2. Blend until smooth and well combined.

3. Add a few ice cubes and blend again to chill the smoothie.

4. Pour into a glass and serve immediately.

Nutrition:

This vibrant smoothie combines the tropical sweetness of mango with the earthy flavor of turmeric and the aromatic freshness of basil. Mango is rich in vitamins A and C. Turmeric adds potential anti-inflammatory properties. Basil adds a burst of flavor and potential health benefits. Almond milk adds creaminess. The nutritional content may vary based on the specific ingredients and optional sweetener used.

Pineapple Ginger Chia Smoothie

Preparation time: 5 minutes

Servings: 1

Ingredients:

- 1 cup chopped pineapple

- 1/2-inch piece of fresh ginger, peeled and grated

- 1 tablespoon chia seeds

- 1 cup coconut water or water

- 1 tablespoon honey or agave syrup (optional, for added sweetness)

- Ice cubes

Directions:

1. In a blender, combine the chopped pineapple, grated ginger, chia seeds, coconut water or water, and sweetener (if using).

2. Blend until smooth and well combined.

3. Add a few ice cubes and blend again to chill the smoothie.

4. Pour into a glass and serve immediately.

Nutrition:

This refreshing smoothie combines the tropical sweetness of pineapple with the spiciness of ginger and the added nutritional benefits of chia seeds. Pineapple provides vitamin C and adds a tropical flavor. Ginger adds a zingy kick and potential digestive benefits. Chia seeds provide fiber and omega-3 fatty acids. Coconut water adds hydration and electrolytes. The nutritional content may vary based on the specific ingredients and optional sweetener used.

Blueberry Pomegranate Smoothie

Preparation time: 5 minutes

Servings: 1

Ingredients:

- 1 cup frozen blueberries

- 1/2 cup pomegranate juice

- 1/2 cup plain Greek yogurt

- 1 tablespoon honey or agave syrup (optional, for added sweetness)

- Ice cubes

Directions:

1. Place the frozen blueberries, pomegranate juice, Greek yogurt, and sweetener (if using) into a blender.

2. Blend until smooth and well combined.

3. Add a few ice cubes and blend again to chill the smoothie.

4. Pour into a glass and serve immediately.

Nutrition:

This antioxidant-rich smoothie combines the sweetness of blueberries with the tanginess of pomegranate. Blueberries are packed with vitamins and minerals. Pomegranate juice adds a burst of flavor and additional antioxidants. Greek yogurt adds creaminess and protein. The nutritional content may vary based on the specific ingredients and optional sweetener used.

Spinach Avocado Cilantro Smoothie

Preparation time: 5 minutes

Servings: 1

Ingredients:

- 1 cup fresh spinach leaves

- 1/2 ripe avocado, peeled and pitted

- 1/4 cup fresh cilantro leaves

- Juice of 1 lime

- 1 cup coconut water or water

- 1 tablespoon honey or agave syrup (optional, for added sweetness)

- Ice cubes

Directions:

1. In a blender, combine the spinach leaves, avocado, cilantro leaves, lime juice, coconut water or water, and sweetener (if using).

2. Blend until smooth and well combined.

3. Add a few ice cubes and blend again to chill the smoothie.

4. Pour into a glass and serve immediately.

Nutrition:

This green smoothie combines the nutrient-rich spinach with the creaminess of avocado and the fresh taste of cilantro. Spinach provides vitamins, minerals, and fiber. Avocado adds healthy fats and a creamy texture. Cilantro adds a unique flavor and potential detoxifying properties. Lime juice adds a tangy twist. The nutritional content may vary based on the specific ingredients and optional sweetener used.

Banana Almond Butter Smoothie

Preparation time: 5 minutes

Servings: 1

Ingredients:

- 1 ripe banana

- 1 tablespoon almond butter

- 1 cup almond milk or any other milk of your choice

- 1 tablespoon honey or agave syrup (optional, for added sweetness)

- Ice cubes

Directions:

1. In a blender, combine the ripe banana, almond butter, almond milk, and sweetener (if using).

2. Blend until smooth and well combined.

3. Add a few ice cubes and blend again to chill the smoothie.

4. Pour into a glass and serve immediately.

Nutrition:

This creamy smoothie combines the sweetness of banana with the nutty flavor of almond butter. Banana provides potassium and natural sweetness. Almond butter adds healthy fats and protein. Almond milk adds creaminess. The nutritional content may vary based on the specific ingredients and optional sweetener used.

Kiwi Kale Ginger Smoothie

Preparation time: 5 minutes

Servings: 1

Ingredients:

- 2 kiwis, peeled and chopped

- 1 cup chopped kale leaves

- 1-inch piece of fresh ginger, peeled and grated

- 1 cup coconut water or water

- 1 tablespoon honey or agave syrup (optional, for added sweetness)

- Ice cubes

Directions:

1. Place the chopped kiwis, kale leaves, grated ginger, coconut water or water, and sweetener (if using) into a blender.

2. Blend until smooth and well combined.

3. Add a few ice cubes and blend again to chill the smoothie.

4. Pour into a glass and serve immediately.

Nutrition:

This vibrant green smoothie combines the tanginess of kiwi with the nutritious kale and the zing of ginger. Kiwi provides vitamin C and fiber. Kale is a nutrient-dense leafy green. Ginger adds a spicy kick and potential digestive benefits. Coconut water adds hydration and electrolytes. The nutritional content may vary based on the specific ingredients and optional sweetener used.

Raspberry Flaxseed Smoothie

Preparation time: 5 minutes

Servings: 1

Ingredients:

- 1 cup frozen raspberries

- 1 tablespoon ground flaxseeds

- 1 cup almond milk or any other milk of your choice

- 1 tablespoon honey or agave syrup (optional, for added sweetness)

- Ice cubes

Directions:

1. Place the frozen raspberries, ground flaxseeds, almond milk, and sweetener (if using) into a blender.

2. Blend until smooth and well combined.

3. Add a few ice cubes and blend again to chill the smoothie.

4. Pour into a glass and serve immediately.

Nutrition:

This antioxidant-rich smoothie combines the sweetness of raspberries with the nutritional benefits of flaxseeds. Raspberries are packed with vitamins and minerals. Flaxseeds provide omega-3 fatty acids and fiber. Almond milk adds creaminess. The nutritional content may vary based on the specific ingredients and optional sweetener used.

Orange Carrot Turmeric Smoothie

Preparation time: 5 minutes

Servings: 1

Ingredients:

- 1 large orange, peeled and segmented

- 1 medium carrot, peeled and chopped

- 1/2 teaspoon ground turmeric

- 1 cup coconut water or water

- 1 tablespoon honey or agave syrup (optional, for added sweetness)

- Ice cubes

Directions:

1. In a blender, combine the orange segments, chopped carrot, ground turmeric, coconut water or water, and sweetener (if using).

2. Blend until smooth and well combined.

3. Add a few ice cubes and blend again to chill the smoothie.

4. Pour into a glass and serve immediately.

Nutrition:

This vibrant orange smoothie combines the citrusy taste of orange with the sweetness of carrot and the earthiness of turmeric. Oranges provide vitamin C and add a refreshing flavor. Carrots are rich in beta-carotene and other nutrients. Turmeric adds potential anti-inflammatory properties. Coconut water adds hydration and electrolytes. The nutritional content may vary based on the specific ingredients and optional sweetener used.

Pear Ginger Cucumber Smoothie

Preparation time: 5 minutes

Servings: 1

Ingredients:

- 1 ripe pear, peeled and chopped

- 1-inch piece of fresh ginger, peeled and grated

- 1/2 small cucumber, peeled and chopped

- 1 cup coconut water or water

- 1 tablespoon honey or agave syrup (optional, for added sweetness)

- Ice cubes

Directions:

1. Place the chopped pear, grated ginger, chopped cucumber, coconut water or water, and sweetener (if using) into a blender.

2. Blend until smooth and well combined.

3. Add a few ice cubes and blend again to chill the smoothie.

4. Pour into a glass and serveimmediately.

Nutrition:

This refreshing smoothie combines the sweetness of pear with the zing of ginger and the hydrating properties of cucumber. Pear provides dietary fiber and vitamins. Ginger adds a spicy kick and potential digestive benefits. Cucumber adds hydration and a cooling effect. Coconut water adds additional hydration and electrolytes. The nutritional content may vary based on the specific ingredients and optional sweetener used.

Watermelon Mint Aloe Vera Smoothie

Preparation time: 5 minutes

Servings: 1

Ingredients:

- 2 cups diced watermelon

- 5-6 fresh mint leaves

- 2 tablespoons aloe vera gel (from a fresh aloe vera leaf or store-bought)

- Juice of 1 lime

- Ice cubes

Directions:

1. In a blender, combine the diced watermelon, mint leaves, aloe vera gel, and lime juice.

2. Blend until smooth and well combined.

3. Add a few ice cubes and blend again to chill the smoothie.

4. Pour into a glass and serve immediately.

Nutrition:

This hydrating smoothie combines the refreshing taste of watermelon with the coolness of mint and the potential benefits of aloe vera. Watermelon is high in water content and provides vitamins A and C. Mint adds a refreshing flavor. Aloe vera may have soothing properties. Lime juice adds a tangy twist. The nutritional content may vary based on the specific ingredients used.

Peach Chamomile Smoothie

Preparation time: 5 minutes

Servings: 1

Ingredients:

- 2 ripe peaches, peeled and pitted

- 1 cup chamomile tea, cooled

- 1/2 cup plain Greek yogurt or any other yogurt of your choice

- 1 tablespoon honey or agave syrup (optional, for added sweetness)

- Ice cubes

Directions:

1. In a blender, combine the peeled and pitted peaches, chamomile tea, Greek yogurt, and sweetener (if using).

2. Blend until smooth and well combined.

3. Add a few ice cubes and blend again to chill the smoothie.

4. Pour into a glass and serve immediately.

Nutrition:

This soothing smoothie combines the sweetness of peaches with the calming effects of chamomile tea. Peaches provide vitamins A and C. Chamomile tea adds a floral and relaxing flavor. Greek yogurt adds creaminess and protein. The nutritional content may vary based on the specific ingredients and optional sweetener used.

Green Apple Celery Smoothie

Preparation time: 5 minutes

Servings: 1

Ingredients:

- 1 green apple, cored and chopped

- 2 stalks celery, chopped

- 1 cup fresh spinach leaves

- 1/2 cup coconut water or water

- Juice of 1/2 lemon

- Ice cubes

Directions:

1. Place the chopped green apple, celery, spinach leaves, coconut water or water, and lemon juice into a blender.

2. Blend until smooth and well combined.

3. Add a few ice cubes and blend again to chill the smoothie.

4. Pour into a glass and serve immediately.

Nutrition:

This green smoothie combines the crispness of green apple with the refreshing taste of celery and the nutritional benefits of spinach. Green apple provides fiber and vitamins. Celery adds hydration and potential detoxifying properties. Spinach provides vitamins, minerals, and fiber. Lemon juice adds a tangy twist. The nutritional content may vary based on the specific ingredients used.

Strawberry Beetroot Smoothie

Preparation time: 5 minutes

Servings: 1

Ingredients:

- 1 cup fresh or frozen strawberries

- 1 small cooked beetroot, peeled and chopped

- 1 cup almond milk or any other milk of your choice

- 1 tablespoon honey or agave syrup (optional, for added sweetness)

- Ice cubes

Directions:

1. In a blender, combine the strawberries, chopped beetroot, almond milk, and sweetener (if using).

2. Blend until smooth and well combined.

3. Add a few ice cubes and blend again to chill the smoothie.

4. Pour into a glass and serve immediately.

Nutrition:

This vibrant smoothie combines the sweetness of strawberries with the earthiness of beetroot. Strawberries are rich in vitamins and antioxidants. Beetroot adds a unique flavor and potential nutritional benefits. Almond milk adds creaminess. The nutritional content may vary based on the specific ingredients and optional sweetener used.

Coconut Blue Spirulina Smoothie

Preparation time: 5 minutes

Servings: 1

Ingredients:

- 1 cup coconut milk

- 1 ripe banana

- 1 teaspoon blue spirulina powder

- 1 tablespoon honey or agave syrup (optional, for added sweetness)

- Ice cubes

Directions:

1. In a blender, combine the coconut milk, ripe banana, blue spirulina powder, and sweetener (if using).

2. Blend until smooth and well combined.

3. Add a few ice cubes and blend again to chill the smoothie.

4. Pour into a glass and serve immediately.

Nutrition:

This vibrant blue smoothie combines the creaminess of coconut milk with the natural sweetness of banana and the added nutritional benefits of blue spirulina. Coconut milk adds richness and healthy fats. Banana providespotassium and natural sweetness. Blue spirulina powder adds a unique color and potential antioxidant properties. The nutritional content may vary based on the specific ingredients and optional sweetener used.

Lemon Ginger Aloe Vera Smoothie

Preparation time: 5 minutes

Servings: 1

Ingredients:

- 1 cup freshly squeezed lemon juice

- 1-inch piece of fresh ginger, peeled and grated

- 2 tablespoons aloe vera gel (from a fresh aloe vera leaf or store-bought)

- 1 tablespoon honey or agave syrup (optional, for added sweetness)

- Ice cubes

Directions:

1. In a blender, combine the freshly squeezed lemon juice, grated ginger, aloe vera gel, and sweetener (if using).

2. Blend until smooth and well combined.

3. Add a few ice cubes and blend again to chill the smoothie.

4. Pour into a glass and serve immediately.

Nutrition:

This invigorating smoothie combines the tanginess of lemon with the warmth of ginger and the potential benefits of aloe vera. Lemon juice provides vitamin C and adds a refreshing flavor. Ginger adds a spicy kick and potential digestive benefits. Aloe vera may have soothing properties. The nutritional content may vary based on the specific ingredients and optional sweetener used.

Spinach Pineapple Mint Smoothie

Preparation time: 5 minutes

Servings: 1

Ingredients:

- 1 cup fresh spinach leaves

- 1 cup chopped pineapple

- 5-6 fresh mint leaves

- 1 cup coconut water or water

- 1 tablespoon honey or agave syrup (optional, for added sweetness)

- Ice cubes

Directions:

1. Place the fresh spinach leaves, chopped pineapple, mint leaves, coconut water or water, and sweetener (if using) into a blender.

2. Blend until smooth and well combined.

3. Add a few ice cubes and blend again to chill the smoothie.

4. Pour into a glass and serve immediately.

Nutrition:

This green smoothie combines the nutrient-rich spinach with the tropical sweetness of pineapple and the refreshing flavor of mint. Spinach provides vitamins, minerals, and fiber. Pineapple adds natural sweetness and contains enzymes that aid digestion. Mint adds a cooling and invigorating taste. Coconut water adds hydration and electrolytes. The nutritional content may vary based on the specific ingredients and optional sweetener used.

Preparation time: 5 minutes

Servings: 1

Ingredients:

- 2 ripe plums, pitted and chopped

- 4-5 fresh basil leaves

- 1 cup almond milk or any other milk of your choice

- 1 tablespoon honey or agave syrup (optional, for added sweetness)

- Ice cubes

Directions:

1. In a blender, combine the chopped plums, basil leaves, almond milk, and sweetener (if using).

2. Blend until smooth and well combined.

3. Add a few ice cubes and blend again to chill the smoothie.

4. Pour into a glass and serve immediately.

Nutrition:

This unique smoothie combines the sweetness of plums with the aromatic flavor of basil. Plums are rich in antioxidants and provide vitamins and fiber. Basil adds a fresh and herbal taste. Almond milk adds creaminess. The nutritional content may vary based on the specific ingredients and optional sweetener used.

Preparation time: 5 minutes

Servings: 1

Ingredients:

- 1 cup fresh or frozen blackberries

- 5-6 fresh mint leaves

- 1 cup coconut milk or any other milk of your choice

- 1 tablespoon honey or agave syrup (optional, for added sweetness)

- Ice cubes

Directions:

1. Place the blackberries, mint leaves, coconut milk, and sweetener (if using) into a blender.

2. Blend until smooth and well combined.

3. Add a few ice cubes and blend again to chill the smoothie.

4. Pour into a glass and serve immediately.

Nutrition:

This refreshing smoothie combines the tangy flavor of blackberries with the cooling taste of mint. Blackberries are rich in antioxidants and provide vitamins and fiber. Mint adds a refreshing and invigorating flavor. Coconut milk adds creaminess and healthy fats. The nutritional content may vary based on the specific ingredients and optional sweetener used.

Apricot Cardamom Smoothie

Preparation time: 5 minutes

Servings: 1

Ingredients:

- 2 ripe apricots, pitted and chopped

- 1 cup almond milk or any other milk of your choice

- 1/2 teaspoon ground cardamom

- 1 tablespoon honey or agave syrup (optional, for added sweetness)

- Ice cubes

Directions:

1. In a blender, combine the chopped apricots, almond milk, ground cardamom, and sweetener (if using).

2. Blend until smooth and well combined.

3. Add a few ice cubes and blend again to chill the smoothie.

4. Pour into a glass and serve immediately.

Nutrition:

This aromatic smoothie combines the sweetnessof apricots with the warm and fragrant flavor of cardamom. Apricots provide vitamins A and C. Cardamom adds a unique and aromatic taste. Almond milk adds creaminess. The nutritional content may vary based on the specific ingredients and optional sweetener used.

Chapter 5:

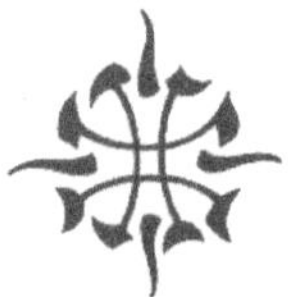

Papaya Banana Coconut Smoothie

Preparation time: 5 minutes

Servings: 1

Ingredients:

- 1 cup ripe papaya, peeled, seeded, and cubed

- 1 ripe banana, peeled and sliced

- 1/2 cup coconut milk

- 1/2 cup coconut water or water

- 1 tablespoon honey or agave syrup (optional, for added sweetness)

- Ice cubes

Directions:

1. In a blender, combine the ripe papaya, banana slices, coconut milk, coconut water or water, and sweetener (if using).

2. Blend until smooth and well combined.

3. Add a few ice cubes and blend again to chill the smoothie.

4. Pour into a glass and serve immediately.

Nutrition:

This tropical smoothie combines the sweetness of papaya with the creaminess of banana and coconut. Papaya provides vitamins A and C, as well as digestive enzymes. Banana adds natural sweetness and potassium. Coconut milk and coconut water add richness and hydration. The nutritional content may vary based on the specific ingredients and optional sweetener used.

Mango Spinach Basil Smoothie

Preparation time: 5 minutes

Servings: 1

Ingredients:

- 1 ripe mango, peeled and cubed

- 1 cup fresh spinach leaves

- 4-5 fresh basil leaves

- 1 cup almond milk or any other milk of your choice

- 1 tablespoon honey or agave syrup (optional, for added sweetness)

- Ice cubes

Directions:

1. Place the cubed mango, spinach leaves, basil leaves, almond milk, and sweetener (if using) into a blender.

2. Blend until smooth and well combined.

3. Add a few ice cubes and blend again to chill the smoothie.

4. Pour into a glass and serve immediately.

Nutrition:

This vibrant green smoothie combines the tropical sweetness of mango with the nutrient-rich spinach and the aromatic flavor of basil. Mango provides vitamins A and C. Spinach adds vitamins, minerals, and fiber. Basil adds a fresh and herbal taste. Almond milk adds creaminess. The nutritional content may vary based on the specific ingredients and optional sweetener used.

Pineapple Turmeric Ginger Smoothie

Preparation time: 5 minutes

Servings: 1

Ingredients:

- 1 cup chopped pineapple

- 1 teaspoon ground turmeric

- 1-inch piece of fresh ginger, peeled and grated

- 1 cup coconut water or water

- Juice of 1/2 lemon

- 1 tablespoon honey or agave syrup (optional, for added sweetness)

- Ice cubes

Directions:

1. In a blender, combine the chopped pineapple, ground turmeric, grated ginger, coconut water or water, lemon juice, and sweetener (if using).

2. Blend until smooth and well combined.

3. Add a few ice cubes and blend again to chill the smoothie.

4. Pour into a glass and serve immediately.

Nutrition:

This vibrant and immune-boosting smoothie combines the tropical sweetness of pineapple with the anti-inflammatory properties of turmeric and the spiciness of ginger. Pineapple provides vitamins and enzymes that aid digestion. Turmeric and ginger add potential anti-inflammatory and antioxidant benefits. Lemon juice adds a tangy twist. The nutritional content may vary based on the specific ingredients and optional sweetener used.

Blueberry Kale Chia Smoothie

Preparation time: 5 minutes

Servings: 1

Ingredients:

- 1 cup fresh or frozen blueberries

- 1 cup chopped kale leaves

- 1 tablespoon chia seeds

- 1 cup almond milk or any other milk of your choice

- 1 tablespoon honey or agave syrup (optional, for added sweetness)

- Ice cubes

Directions:

1. Place the blueberries, kale leaves, chia seeds, almond milk, and sweetener (if using) into a blender.

2. Blend until smooth and well combined.

3. Add a few ice cubes and blend again to chill the smoothie.

4. Pour into a glass and serve immediately.

Nutrition:

This antioxidant-rich smoothie combines the sweetness of blueberries with the nutritional benefits of kale and chia seeds. Blueberries are packed with vitamins and antioxidants. Kale provides vitamins, minerals, and fiber. Chia seeds add omega-3 fatty acids and fiber. Almond milk adds creaminess. The nutritional content may vary based on the specific ingredients and optional sweetener used.

Avocado Cucumber Mint Smoothie

Preparation time: 5 minutes

Servings: 1

Ingredients:

- 1/2 ripe avocado, peeled and pitted

- 1/2 medium cucumber, peeled and chopped

- 5-6 fresh mint leaves

- Juice of 1/2 lime

- 1 cup coconut water or water

- Ice cubes

Directions:

1. In a blender, combine the ripe avocado, chopped cucumber, mint leaves, lime juice, coconut water or water.

2. Blend until smooth and well combined.

3. Add a few ice cubes and blend again to chill the smoothie.

4. Pour into a glass and serve immediately.

Nutrition:

This refreshing smoothie combines the creamy texture of avocado with the cooling flavors of cucumber and mint. Avocado provides healthy fats and vitamins. Cucumber adds hydration and a refreshing taste. Mint adds a cooling and invigorating flavor. Lime juice adds a tangy twist. The nutritional content may vary based on the specific ingredients used.

Kiwi Flaxseed Smoothie

Preparation time: 5 minutes

Servings: 1

Ingredients:

- 2 ripe kiwis, peeled and sliced

- 1 tablespoon flaxseeds

- 1 cup almond milk or any other milk of your choice

- 1 tablespoon honey or agave syrup (optional, for added sweetness)

- Ice cubes

Directions:

1. In a blender, combine the sliced kiwis, flaxseeds, almond milk, and sweetener (if using).

2. Blend until smooth and well combined.

3. Add a few ice cubes and blend again to chill the smoothie.

4. Pour into a glass and serve immediately.

Nutrition:

This refreshing smoothie combines the vibrant flavor of kiwi with the nutritional benefits of flaxseeds. Kiwi provides vitamin C and dietary fiber. Flaxseeds are a great source of omega-3 fatty acids and fiber. Almond milk adds creaminess. The nutritional content may vary based on the specific ingredients and optional sweetener used.

Raspberry Coconut Water Smoothie

Preparation time: 5 minutes

Servings: 1

Ingredients:

- 1 cup fresh or frozen raspberries

- 1 cup coconut water

- 1 tablespoon honey or agave syrup (optional, for added sweetness)

- Ice cubes

Directions:

1. Place the raspberries, coconut water, and sweetener (if using) into a blender.

2. Blend until smooth and well combined.

3. Add a few ice cubes and blend again to chill the smoothie.

4. Pour into a glass and serve immediately.

Nutrition:

This refreshing and hydrating smoothie combines the tartness of raspberries with the electrolyte-rich coconut water. Raspberries are rich in antioxidants and vitamins. Coconut water helps to replenish electrolytes and provides natural sweetness. The nutritional content may vary based on the specific ingredients and optional sweetener used.

Preparation time: 5 minutes

Servings: 1

Ingredients:

- 1 medium orange, peeled and segmented

- 1 medium carrot, peeled and chopped

- 1 small beetroot, peeled and chopped

- 1 cup coconut water or water

- 1 tablespoon honey or agave syrup (optional, for added sweetness)

- Ice cubes

Directions:

1. In a blender, combine the orange segments, chopped carrot, chopped beetroot, coconut water or water, and sweetener (if using).

2. Blend until smooth and well combined.

3. Add a few ice cubes and blend again to chill the smoothie.

4. Pour into a glass and serve immediately.

Nutrition:

This vibrant and nutrient-rich smoothie combines the sweetness of orange with the earthy flavors of carrot and beetroot. Oranges provide vitamin C and natural sweetness. Carrots are rich in vitamins and beta-carotene.

Beetroot adds antioxidants and potential blood pressure benefits. Coconut water adds hydration and electrolytes. The nutritional content may vary based on the specific ingredients and optional sweetener used.

Pear Celery Ginger Smoothie

Preparation time: 5 minutes

Servings: 1

Ingredients:

- 1 ripe pear, peeled, cored, and chopped

- 1 stalk celery, chopped

- 1-inch piece of fresh ginger, peeled and grated

- 1 cup almond milk or any other milk of your choice

- 1 tablespoon honey or agave syrup (optional, for added sweetness)

- Ice cubes

Directions:

1. Place the chopped pear, celery, grated ginger, almond milk, and sweetener (if using) into a blender.

2. Blend until smooth and well combined.

3. Add a few ice cubes and blend again to chill the smoothie.

4. Pour into a glass and serve immediately.

Nutrition:

This refreshing and fiber-rich smoothie combines the sweetness of pear with the crispness of celery and the spiciness of ginger. Pears provide vitamins, minerals, and dietary fiber. Celery adds hydration and a fresh taste. Ginger adds a spicy kick and potential digestive benefits. Almond milk adds creaminess. The nutritional content may vary based on the specific ingredients and optional sweetener used.

Watermelon Mint Lime Smoothie

Preparation time: 5 minutes

Servings: 1

Ingredients:

- 2 cups cubed seedless watermelon

- 5-6 fresh mint leaves

- Juice of 1 lime

- 1 cup coconut water or water

- Ice cubes

Directions:

1. In a blender, combine the cubed watermelon, mint leaves, lime juice, and coconut water or water.

2. Blend until smooth and well combined.

3. Add a few ice cubes and blend again to chill the smoothie.

4. Pour into a glass and serve immediately.

Nutrition:

This hydrating and refreshing smoothie combines the sweetness of watermelon with the cooling flavors of mint and lime. Watermelon is rich in vitamins A and C, and it provides hydration due to its high water content. Mint adds a fresh and cooling taste, while lime juice adds a tangy twist. Coconut water adds electrolytes and natural sweetness. The nutritional content may vary based on the specific ingredients used.

Peach Turmeric Cilantro Smoothie

Preparation time: 5 minutes

Servings: 1

Ingredients:

- 1 ripe peach, peeled, pitted, and sliced

- 1/2 teaspoon ground turmeric

- Small handful of fresh cilantro leaves

- 1 cup coconut water or water

- 1 tablespoon honey or agave syrup (optional, for added sweetness)

- Ice cubes

Directions:

1. In a blender, combine the sliced peach, ground turmeric, cilantro leaves, coconut water or water, and sweetener (if using).

2. Blend until smooth and well combined.

3. Add a few ice cubes and blend again to chill the smoothie.

4. Pour into a glass and serve immediately.

Nutrition:

This unique smoothie combines the sweetness of peach with the anti-inflammatory properties of turmeric and the refreshing taste of cilantro. Peaches are rich in vitamins and antioxidants. Turmeric adds potential anti-inflammatory benefits. Cilantro adds a fresh and herbal taste. Coconut water provides hydration and natural sweetness. The nutritional content may vary based on the specific ingredients and optional sweetener used.

Green Apple Spinach Ginger Smoothie

Preparation time: 5 minutes

Servings: 1

Ingredients:

- 1 medium green apple, cored and chopped

- 1 cup fresh spinach leaves

- 1-inch piece of fresh ginger, peeled and grated

- 1 cup almond milk or any other milk of your choice

- 1 tablespoon honey or agave syrup (optional, for added sweetness)

- Ice cubes

Directions:

1. Place the chopped green apple, spinach leaves, grated ginger, almond milk, and sweetener (if using) into a blender.

2. Blend until smooth and well combined.

3. Add a few ice cubes and blend again to chill the smoothie.

4. Pour into a glass and serve immediately.

Nutrition:

This refreshing and nutrient-rich smoothie combines the crispness of green apple with the nutritional benefits of spinach and the spiciness of ginger. Green apples provide vitamins and dietary fiber. Spinach adds vitamins, minerals, and fiber. Ginger adds a spicy kick and potential digestive benefits. Almond milk adds creaminess. The nutritional content may vary based on the specific ingredients and optional sweetener used.

Strawberry Pineapple Mint Smoothie

Preparation time: 5 minutes

Servings: 1

Ingredients:

- 1 cup fresh or frozen strawberries

- 1 cup chopped pineapple

- Small handful of fresh mint leaves

- 1 cup coconut water or water

- 1 tablespoon honey or agave syrup (optional, for added sweetness)

- Ice cubes

Directions:

1. In a blender, combine the strawberries, chopped pineapple, mint leaves, coconut water or water, and sweetener (if using).

2. Blend until smooth and well combined.

3. Add a few ice cubes and blend again to chill the smoothie.

4. Pour into a glass and serve immediately.

Nutrition:

This tropical and refreshing smoothie combines the sweetness of strawberries with the tanginess of pineapple and the cooling flavors of mint. Strawberries are rich in vitamins and antioxidants. Pineapple provides vitamins and enzymes that aid digestion. Mint adds a fresh and cooling taste. Coconut water adds hydration and natural sweetness. The nutritional content may vary based on the specific ingredients and optional sweetener used.

Coconut Blueberry Smoothie

Preparation time: 5 minutes

Servings: 1

Ingredients:

- 1 cup fresh or frozen blueberries

- 1/2 cup coconut milk

- 1/2 cup coconut water or water

- 1 tablespoon honey or agave syrup (optional, for added sweetness)

- Ice cubes

Directions:

1. Place the blueberries, coconut milk, coconut water or water, and sweetener (if using) into a blender.

2. Blend until smooth and well combined.

3. Add a few ice cubes and blend again to chill the smoothie.

4. Pour into a glass and serve immediately.

Nutrition:

This creamy and antioxidant-rich smoothie combines the sweetness of blueberries with the richness of coconut. Blueberries are packed with vitamins and antioxidants. Coconut milk adds creaminess and healthy fats. Coconut water provides hydration and natural sweetness. The nutritional content may vary based on the specific ingredients and optional sweetener used.

Lemon Ginger Spinach Smoothie

Preparation time: 5 minutes

Servings: 1

Ingredients:

- Juice of 1 lemon

- 1-inch piece of fresh ginger, peeled and grated

- 1 cup fresh spinach leaves

- 1 cup almond milk or any other milk of your choice

- 1 tablespoon honey or agave syrup (optional, for added sweetness)

- Ice cubes

Directions:

1. In a blender, combine the lemon juice, grated ginger, spinach leaves, almond milk, and sweetener (if using).

2. Blend until smooth and well combined.

3. Add a few ice cubes and blend again to chill the smoothie.

4. Pour into a glass and serve immediately.

Nutrition:

This zesty and energizing smoothie combines the tanginess of lemon with the spiciness of ginger and the nutritional benefits of spinach. Lemons are rich in vitamin C and provide a refreshing taste. Ginger adds a spicy kick and potential digestive benefits. Spinach adds vitamins, minerals, and fiber. Almond milk adds creaminess. The nutritional content may vary based on the specific ingredients and optional sweetener used.

Spinach Pineapple Coconut Smoothie

Preparation time: 5 minutes

Servings: 1

Ingredients:

- 1 cup fresh spinach leaves

- 1 cup chopped pineapple

- 1/2 cup coconut milk

- 1/2 cup coconut water or water

- 1 tablespoon honey or agave syrup (optional, for added sweetness)

- Ice cubes

Directions:

1. Place the spinach leaves, chopped pineapple, coconut milk, coconut water or water, and sweetener (if using) into a blender.

2. Blend until smooth and well combined.

3. Add a few ice cubes and blend again to chill the smoothie.

4. Pour into a glass and serve immediately.

Nutrition:

This tropical and nutritious smoothie combines the leafy goodness of spinach with the sweetness and tanginess of pineapple and the richness of coconut. Spinach provides vitamins, minerals, and fiber. Pineapple adds vitamins and enzymes that aid digestion. Coconut milk adds creaminess and healthy fats. Coconut water provides hydration and natural sweetness. The nutritional content may vary based on the specific ingredients and optional sweetener used.

Plum Kiwi Basil Smoothie

Preparation time: 5 minutes

Servings: 1

Ingredients:

- 2 ripe plums, pitted and chopped

- 2 ripe kiwis, peeled and chopped

- Small handful of fresh basil leaves

- 1 cup coconut water or water

- 1 tablespoon honey or agave syrup (optional, for added sweetness)

- Ice cubes

Directions:

1. In a blender, combine the chopped plums, chopped kiwis, basil leaves, coconut water or water, and sweetener (if using).

2. Blend until smooth and well combined.

3. Add a few ice cubes and blend again to chill the smoothie.

4. Pour into a glass and serve immediately.

Nutrition:

This unique and flavorful smoothie combines the sweetness of plums with the tartness of kiwis and the fresh taste of basil. Plums are rich in vitamins and antioxidants. Kiwis provide vitamin C and dietary fiber. Basil adds an aromatic and herbal touch. Coconut water adds hydration and natural sweetness. The nutritional content may vary based on the specific ingredients and optional sweetener used.

Blackberry Pear Ginger Smoothie

Preparation time: 5 minutes

Servings: 1

Ingredients:

- 1 cup fresh blackberries

- 1 ripe pear, peeled, cored, and chopped

- 1-inch piece of fresh ginger, peeled and grated

- 1 cup almond milk or any other milk of your choice

- 1 tablespoon honey or agave syrup (optional, for added sweetness)

- Ice cubes

Directions:

1. In a blender, combine the blackberries, chopped pear, grated ginger, almond milk, and sweetener (if using).

2. Blend until smooth and well combined.

3. Add a few ice cubes and blend again to chill the smoothie.

4. Pour into a glass and serve immediately.

Nutrition:

This antioxidant-rich smoothie combines the sweet and tangy flavors of blackberries and pear with the spiciness of ginger. Blackberries are packed with vitamins and antioxidants. Pears provide vitamins, minerals, and dietary fiber. Ginger adds a spicy kick and potential digestive benefits. Almond milk adds creaminess. The nutritional content may vary based on the specific ingredients and optional sweetener used.

Apricot Mango Cilantro Smoothie

Preparation time: 5 minutes

Servings: 1

Ingredients:

- 2 ripe apricots, pitted and chopped

- 1 ripe mango, peeled, pitted, and chopped

- Small handful of fresh cilantro leaves

- 1 cup coconut water or water

- 1 tablespoon honey or agave syrup (optional, for added sweetness)

- Ice cubes

Directions:

1. Place the chopped apricots, chopped mango, cilantro leaves, coconut water or water, and sweetener (if using) into a blender.

2. Blend until smooth and well combined.

3. Add a few ice cubes and blend again to chill the smoothie.

4. Pour into a glass and serve immediately.

Nutrition:

This tropical and refreshing smoothie combines the sweetness of apricots and mango with the fresh taste of cilantro. Apricots are rich in vitamins and antioxidants. Mango provides vitamins A and C, as well as natural sweetness. Cilantro adds an herbal touch. Coconut water adds hydration and natural sweetness. The nutritional content may vary based on the specific ingredients and optional sweetener used.

Papaya Turmeric Mint Smoothie

Preparation time: 5 minutes

Servings: 1

Ingredients:

- 1 cup ripe papaya, peeled, seeded, and chopped

- 1/2 teaspoon ground turmeric

- Small handful of fresh mint leaves

- 1 cup coconut water or water

- 1 tablespoon honey or agave syrup (optional, foradded sweetness)

- Ice cubes

Directions:

1. In a blender, combine the chopped papaya, ground turmeric, mint leaves, coconut water or water, and sweetener (if using).

2. Blend until smooth and well combined.

3. Add a few ice cubes and blend again to chill the smoothie.

4. Pour into a glass and serve immediately.

Nutrition:

This vibrant and tropical smoothie combines the sweetness of papaya with the anti-inflammatory properties of turmeric and the refreshing taste of mint. Papaya is rich in vitamins A and C, as well as digestive enzymes. Turmeric adds potential anti-inflammatory benefits. Mint adds a fresh and cooling taste. Coconut water adds hydration and natural sweetness. The nutritional content may vary based on the specific ingredients and optional sweetener used.

Chapter 6:

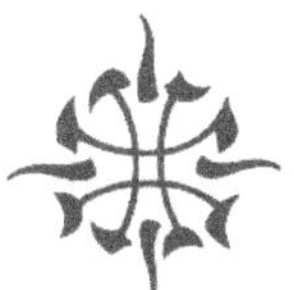

CONCLUSION: NURTURING YOUR GUT HEALTH JOURNEY

Recapitulation of Gut Health Importance

Gut health refers to the well-being of the gastrointestinal system, which includes the stomach, small intestine, and large intestine. A healthy gut is crucial for overall well-being as it plays a significant role in digestion, nutrient absorption, immune function, and even mental health.

The gut is home to trillions of microorganisms, collectively known as the gut microbiota or gut flora. These beneficial bacteria help break down food, produce essential nutrients, and support a strong immune system. When the balance of gut bacteria is disrupted, it can lead to various health issues, including digestive problems, inflammation, and a weakened immune system.

Maintaining a healthy gut involves adopting a balanced and nutritious diet, managing stress levels, getting regular exercise, and getting enough sleep. Including gut-friendly foods in your diet, such as fiber-rich fruits and vegetables, fermented foods, and probiotics, can also support optimal gut health.

The Role of Smoothies in Supporting Gut Health

Smoothies can be an excellent addition to a gut-healthy diet. They offer several benefits that support digestive health:

a. Nutrient-dense ingredients: Smoothies can be packed with fruits, vegetables, and other nutritious ingredients that provide essential vitamins, minerals, and antioxidants. These nutrients support overall health and help nourish the gut.

b. Fiber content: Many smoothie ingredients, such as fruits, vegetables, and seeds, are excellent sources of dietary fiber. Fiber plays a crucial role in maintaining regular bowel movements, supporting healthy digestion, and promoting the growth of beneficial gut bacteria.

c. Hydration: Smoothies often contain hydrating ingredients like coconut water, watermelon, or cucumber, which help maintain proper hydration levels. Good hydration is essential for optimal digestion and overall gut health.

d. Probiotic potential: Adding probiotic-rich ingredients like yogurt, kefir, or fermented foods to your smoothies can introduce beneficial bacteria to your gut. Probiotics help restore the balance of gut flora and support a healthy digestive system.

e. Easy to digest: Blending ingredients into a smoothie can help break them down, making it easier for your body to digest and absorb the nutrients. This can be especially beneficial for individuals with digestive issues or those who have difficulty chewing certain foods.

Tips for Incorporating Gut-Healing Smoothies into Your Routine

Here are some tips to help you incorporate gut-healing smoothies into your daily routine:

a. Choose gut-friendly ingredients: Include fruits, vegetables, leafy greens, seeds, and probiotic-rich foods like yogurt or kefir in your smoothies. These ingredients provide fiber, vitamins, minerals, and beneficial bacteria that support gut health.

b. Focus on fiber: Aim to incorporate fiber-rich ingredients like berries, apples, pears, leafy greens, chia seeds, flaxseeds, or oats into your smoothies. Fiber promotes healthy digestion and feeds beneficial gut bacteria.

c. Experiment with herbs and spices: Add gut-friendly herbs and spices like ginger, mint, basil, turmeric, or cinnamon to your smoothies. These ingredients can have anti-inflammatory and digestive benefits.

d. Include healthy fats: Adding sources of healthy fats like avocado, coconut milk, or nut butter to your smoothies can enhance nutrient absorption and provide satiety.

e. Avoid excessive added sugars: Be mindful of the amount of added sugars in your smoothies. Too much sugar can disrupt gut health. Instead, use natural sweeteners like honey or opt for naturally sweet fruits.

f. Consider food sensitivities: If you have known food sensitivities or intolerances, avoid ingredients that trigger symptoms. Customize your smoothies based on your individual needs and preferences.

g. Make it a regular habit: Aim to have a gut-healing smoothie as part of your daily routine. Consistency is key when it comes to reaping the benefits of gut-friendly foods.

Remember that while smoothies can be a valuable addition to a gut-healthy diet, they should not replace whole foods or a balanced diet. It's always best to consult with a healthcare professional or registered dietitian for personalized advice, especially if you have specific health concerns or conditions related to gut health.

Maintaining long-term gut health involves adopting healthy lifestyle habits and incorporating gut-friendly practices into your daily routine. Here are some strategies to consider:

a. Balanced and varied diet: Focus on consuming a diverse range of fruits, vegetables, whole grains, lean proteins, and healthy fats. Include fiber-rich foods and fermented foods like yogurt, sauerkraut, or kefir to promote a healthy gut microbiota.

b. Stay hydrated: Drink plenty of water throughout the day to support proper digestion and maintain optimal hydration levels.

c. Manage stress: Chronic stress can negatively impact gut health. Practice stress management techniques such as deep breathing, meditation, yoga, or engaging in hobbies and activities you enjoy.

d. Prioritize sleep: Aim for quality sleep to support overall health, including gut health. Create a consistent sleep schedule, establish a relaxing bedtime routine, and create a sleep-friendly environment.

e. Regular exercise: Engage in regular physical activity, as it can help regulate digestion, reduce stress, and support overall well-being. Find activities you enjoy and make them a regular part of your routine.

f. Limit processed foods and additives: Minimize the consumption of processed foods, refined sugars, artificial sweeteners, and additives as they can negatively affect gut health. Opt for whole, minimally processed foods whenever possible.

g. Avoid excessive antibiotic use: Antibiotics can disrupt the balance of gut bacteria. Use antibiotics only when necessary and follow your healthcare provider's instructions.

h. Seek professional guidance: If you have persistent digestive issues or concerns about your gut health, consult with a healthcare professional or registered dietitian who specializes in gut health. They can provide personalized guidance and recommendations based on your specific needs.

Taking steps to improve and maintain your gut health is an accomplishment worth celebrating. Here are some ways to celebrate your gut health success:

a. Reflect on your progress: Take a moment to reflect on how far you've come in your gut health journey. Acknowledge the positive changes you've made and the improvements you've experienced.

b. Share your success: Share your gut health journey with friends, family, or a supportive community. You might inspire others to prioritize their gut health as well.

c. Treat yourself: Treat yourself to something special as a reward for your commitment to gut health. It could be a relaxing spa day, a healthy meal at your favorite restaurant, or a new kitchen gadget to continue experimenting with gut-friendly recipes.

d. Maintain gratitude: Cultivate an attitude of gratitude for your body's resilience and its ability to heal and adapt. Appreciate the progress you've made and the positive impact it has had on your overall well-being.

e. Set new goals: Set new goals to continue improving your gut health. Whether it's trying new gut-healing recipes, exploring different stress management techniques, or incorporating other healthy habits into your routine, keep challenging yourself to maintain and enhance your gut health.

Final Thoughts and Encouragement

Prioritizing gut health is a long-term journey that requires consistency and mindfulness. It's important to remember that everyone's gut health is unique, and what works for one person may not work for another. Be patient with yourself and embrace the process of finding what works best for your body.

Celebrate the small victories along the way, as even small changes can have a significant impact on your gut health and overall well-being. Stay committed to a balanced and healthy lifestyle, and remember that progress is often gradual.

If you encounter challenges or setbacks, don't get discouraged. Use them as opportunities to learn and adjust your approach. Remember to seek support from healthcare professionals or registered dietitians who can provide personalized guidance and support.

With dedication, awareness, and a focus on nurturing your gut, you can achieve and maintain optimal gut health, leading to improved digestion, enhanced immunity, and overall vitality.